Vegan Diet

Plant-Based Diet for Weight Loss and Energy in 30 days

(A Quick and Easy Guide to Making Amazing Meals and Snacks for Everyone)

Sidney Griffin

Published by Robert Satterfield Publishing House

© **Sidney Griffin**

All Rights Reserved

Vegan Diet Recipes: Plant-Based Diet for Weight Loss and Energy in 30 days (A Quick and Easy Guide to Making Amazing Meals and Snacks for Everyone)

ISBN 978-1-989787-09-0

All rights reserved. No part of this guide may be reproduced in any form without permission in writing from the publisher except in the case of brief quotations embodied in critical articles or reviews.

Legal & Disclaimer

The information contained in this book is not designed to replace or take the place of any form of medicine or professional medical advice. The information in this book has been provided for educational and entertainment purposes only.

The information contained in this book has been compiled from sources deemed reliable, and it is accurate to the best of the Author's knowledge; however, the Author cannot guarantee its accuracy and validity and cannot be held liable for any errors or omissions. Changes are periodically made to this book. You must consult your doctor or get professional medical advice before using any of the suggested remedies, techniques, or information in this book.

TABLE OF CONTENT

Part 1 1

Introduction 2

Blueberry Banana Muffins *Yields 12 Muffins* 2

Strawberry Shortcake Pancakes *Yields 6 Pancakes* 3

Garden Frittata *Yields 3-4* 6

Peach Pie Oatmeal *Yields 1 Serving* 8

Peanut Butter Banana Toast *Yields 2 Servings* 9

Cinnamon Blackberry Quinoa 10

Peach Balsamic Wrap Yields 2 Servings 12

Over The Top Green Salad *Yields 2 Servings* 14

Pear Salad Yields 1 Serving... 16

Cauliflower Soup Yields 6-8 Servings 18

Dinner 20

Chinese Sweet Potatoes... 20

Black Bean Burger 22

Broccoli Tofu Stir-Fry... 24

Roasted Potato Bowl *Yields 3 Servings* 26

Sweet Potato Bean Chili 28

Veggie And Chimichurri Hash *Yields 3 Servings* 29

Lemon Garlic Brussel Sprouts 31

Sweet Potato Patties *Yields 12 Patties* 31

Cheesy Acorn Alfredo 33

Lentil Burgers Yield 8 Small Burgers 34

Snacks And Desserts 35

Apple Pie And Whipped Cream 36

Cranberry And Seed Granola Bars *Yields 10-12 Bars* 39

Citrus Granola Parfait *Yields 4 Servings* 41

Potato Pudding Yields 3 Servings 42

Conclusion 44

Part 2 45

Introduction 46

Fudge Brownies 47

Vanilla Ice Cream 49

Choco Peanut Butter Ice Cream 50

Mint Chocolate Chip Ice Cream 51

Maple Walnut Ice Cream 52

Salted Bourbon Caramel Ice Cream 53

Chocolate Chip Cookies... 55

Peanut Butter Cookies 56

Dark Chocolate Macaroons.. 58

Snickerdoodles 59

Gingerbread Cookies... 61

Shortbread Cookies... 63

Chewy Molasses Cookies 64

Chocolate-Covered Frozen Banana Bites.............................. 66

Peanut Butter Chocolate Balls 67

Dark Chocolate Truffles... 69

Cinnamon Rolls 70

Vanilla Cupcakes 72

Red Velvet Cupcakes With Cream Cheese Frosting 74

Chocolate Cake 77

Cinnamon Coffee Cake 79

Pineapple Upside-Down Cake 81

Lemon Cake 83

Carrot Cake 84

Red Velvet Brownies 87

Blueberry Crisp 88

Peach Cobbler 90

Chocolate Mousse 91

Tiramisu 92

Chocolate Açaí Bowl 95

Banana Pudding 96

Chocolate Dessert Shake 97

Vanilla Cashew Shake 98

Pumpkin Pie 99

Deep Dish Apple Pie 101

Sweet Potato Pie 104

Pecan Pie 106

About The Author 110

Part 1

Introduction

Active bodies make a lot of demands from the food that is fed to it. Muscle needs to be built, fat needs to remain minimal, energy needs boosting. But is it possible to get everything that a body requires and cut animal products at the same time?

Are vegans forced into raw food diets or are there ways to enjoy plant based foods without sacrificing taste? The answer to all of these questions is yes, it is possible, and your body and mind will thank you for it.

Blueberry Banana Muffins *yields 12 muffins*

Ingredients
2 1/3 cups oat flour
3 tsp baking powder
½ tsp salt
½ cup lemon juice
1/2 cup almond milk
2 bananas, ripe enough for mashing

1 tsp chia seeds
½ tsp flax seeds
½ cup maple syrup
1 cup blueberries
½ cup sliced almonds
1 tbsp coconut oil
Pinch of ginger (optional)

Directions

Preheat oven to 350. Line muffin tin and spray with non-stick spray. Blend together oat flour, salt, and baking powder in a large bowl. In a blender, blend lemon juice, almond milk, bananas, chia seeds, flax seeds, and syrup on low speed until mixture is smooth. Add to dry ingredients and stir until it forms a soft batter. Fold in remaining ingredients until mixed well. Fill muffin cups until they are 2/3 full and bake for 15-20 minutes, until they are browned on top and a toothpick comes out clean. Cool for 10 minutes and serve!

Strawberry Shortcake Pancakes *yields 6 pancakes*

Ingredients

1 ¼ cup whole wheat flour
½ cup shredded coconut
1 tsp baking powder
½ tsp nutmeg
½ tsp allspice
½ tsp cinnamon
Pinch of kosher salt
¾ cup coconut milk
½ tsp vanilla extract
1 tbsp maple syrup
¾ cup warm water
Coconut oil for frying
6 strawberries and one frozen banana, processed into soft serve

*Optional: Sliced banana and strawberries

Directions

Preheat skillet over medium heat and add a small amount of coconut oil. Mix together flour, shredded coconut, baking soda, baking powder, nutmeg, allspice, cinnamon, and salt in a medium bowl. In a separate bowl, whisk coconut milk, water, vanilla, and syrup. Add to dry ingredients. Stir well until smooth and no clumps are present. Pour ¼ cup per pancake onto skillet. Cook until edges begin to appear dry and bubbles appear on surface. Flip and cook on underside only until lightly browned. When serving, place a heaping spoonful of strawberry banana soft serve on top and sliced bananas and strawberries if desired.

The great thing about these pancakes, is you can add whatever garnishes you'd like, such as blueberries and sliced almonds. Have fun with them!

Garden Frittata *yields 3-4*

Ingredients

1 russet potato, peeled and thinly sliced
7 ounces soft silken tofu
2 tbsp vegan margarine
3 tbsp arrowroot
1 tsp baking powder
1 tsp sea salt
½ tsp black pepper
½ tsp turmeric
½ tsp onion powder
½ tsp garlic powder
2 tbsp olive oil
1 onion, chopped
1 zucchini, shredded
1 small tomato, sliced

Directions

Preheat oven to broil. Boil slices of potato until they are tender and then drain. Blend tofu, margarine, arrowroot, baking powder, salt, pepper, turmeric, onion powder, and garlic powder until well blended. Heat oil over medium heat in 9 inch oven-safe skillet. Cook onions until soft and browned. Add shredded zucchini and cooked potatoes and allow to cook for several minutes. Add tofu mixture and lower heat to medium-low. Turn over mixture several times to ensure that the vegetables are completely covered. Smooth mixture and place tomato slices on top. Allow to cook for 15 minutes. Place skillet in oven and broil for 3-5 minutes or until the top has begun to brown. Allow to cool for 15-20 minutes.

*Optional: Garnish with basil leaves

Peach Pie Oatmeal *yields 1 serving*

Ingredients

3/3 cup oats
1 ½ cups water
¼ tsp salt
1 tsp vanilla extract
1 cup diced peaches (throw in some diced nectarines if you'd like)
2 tbsp orange juice
½ tsp cinnamon
¼ sliced banana
1 tsp chia seeds
½ cup soy or almond milk
2 tbsp chopped nuts (pecans or walnuts)

Directions

In a saucepan, cook oats in water with salt, ¼ tsp cinnamon and vanilla. Once oats are fully cooked, add to bowl and stir in desired amount of milk and chia seeds. If desired, add sweetener, such as agave nectar over top of oatmeal. Stir together diced peaches with remaining cinnamon and orange juice and spoon over top.

Peanut Butter Banana Toast *yields 2 servings*

Ingredients

4 slices bread (toasted)
4 tbsp peanut butter (almond butter can also be used)
2 bananas (ripe)
1 tsp syrup or agave nectar
2 tsp cinnamon

Directions

Mash bananas, peanut butter, cinnamon and sweetener. Spread on toast.

*optional: add seeds, chopped nuts or even sliced fruit on top

Cinnamon Blackberry Quinoa

Yields 4 servings

Ingredients

1 cup almond or soy milk
1 cup water
1 cup quinoa, rinsed
2 cups black or blueberries
½ tsp cinnamon
1/3 cup chopped, toasted pecans or walnuts
4 tsp agave nectar or honey

Directions

Stir together water, milk, and quinoa in saucepan and boil over high heat. Reduce to medium-low, cover, and simmer until most liquid is absorbed (about 15 minutes). Remove from heat and allow to stand for several minutes before adding berries and cinnamon. Serve with nuts and sweetener drizzled over top.

Lunch

The time for sandwiches with cheap, supermarket lunchmeat, a burger at the fast food joint around the corner, or even just a quick snack while you run from one meeting to another is over. You're in the middle of your busy afternoon and you need something to pick you up and keep you going. Wraps keep better than soggy bread so preparing them the morning of will make for a quick grab when lunch rolls around and you're on the run. Soups and chowders can be made the night before and quickly warmed. Add a quick snack such as some raw carrots, an apple with peanut butter, or chunks of fruit and you have an ideal meal to leave you motivated.

Peach Balsamic Wrap yields 2 servings

Ingredients

2 large wraps
2 small, sliced peaches
1 sliced avocado
Fresh basil, chopped
1 tsp lemon juice or orange juice
Handful of spinach
4 tbsp extra virgin olive oil
4 tbsp balsamic vinegar
Pinch of salt
Pinch of black pepper
2 tsp Dijon mustard
1 tbsp chopped onion

Directions

Toss peaches and avocado with lemon or orange juice. Blend olive oil, vinegar, salt, pepper, mustard, and chopped onion in food processor to make balsamic dressing. Warm wraps over stove top for only a few seconds per side or just toss in the oven for a couple of minutes. Stir together peach mixture, basil, with a small amount of dressing. Fill wraps with mixture, adding in spinach, and add a bit more dressing over top. Roll wrap and allow to cool before serving.

*Optional: Add in any other desired vegetables or greens such as tomatoes, cucumbers, or even cooked asparagus

Over the Top Green Salad *yields 2 servings*

Ingredients

2 cups thinly chopped green chard
2 cups thinly chopped kale
½ cup cooked chick peas
½ cup diced avocado
1/8 tsp lemon zest
1 peeled Satsuma orange
1 ½ tbsp. creamy tahini
1 tbsp apple cider vinegar
1 tsp lemon juice
3 tsp maple syrup
1 tsp black pepper
Pinch of salt
Pinch of cayenne

Directions

Stir together greens and lemon zest. Rinse peas under hot water and rinse in cold water. Remove skins and toast if desired. Mix together avocado and greens. Whisk together tahini, vinegar, lemon juice, syrup, pepper, salt, and cayenne and toss with salad mixture. Fold peas into salad and serve, topped with orange slices.

*Optional: Drizzle Omega rich oil over salad mixture

Pear Salad yields 1 serving

Ingredients

2 bunches kale, stems removed
2 medium pears, sliced
½ cup chopped pecans
½ cup Extra Virgin olive oil
1 shallot
2 tbsp Dijon mustard
2 tbsp Champagne vinegar
1 tbsp lemon juice
1/8 tsp sea salt
1 tbsp honey
1 crushed garlic clove
Coconut oil
Pinch of salt
Pinch of black pepper

Directions

Combine olive oil, shallot, vinegar, lemon juice, garlic, mustard, honey and sea salt to create dressing. Lightly oil sauté pan with coconut oil and cook kale in small batches over medium low heat until kale is soft. Toss in dressing, serve on plate topped with pears, pecans, salt and pepper.

Cauliflower Soup yields 6-8 servings

Ingredients

2 tbsp extra-virgin olive oil
2 medium thinly sliced white onions
1/2 tsp kosher salt
4 cloves minced garlic
1 large head of cauliflower, trimmed and cut
4 1/2 cups vegetable broth (or water)
1/2 tsp coriander
1/2 tsp turmeric
1 1/4 tsp cumin
1 cup coconut milk
Black pepper
1/4 cup cashew halves
1/4 cup finely chopped Italian parsley
Red chili pepper flakes

Directions

In large pot over medium heat, heat oil until simmering. Cook onions and 1/4 tsp salt until onions are translucent. Reduce heat to low and add garlic. Cook for two minutes. Add cauliflower, broth, coriander, turmeric, cumin, and remaining salt. Boil over medium high head then reduce to low. Simmer about 15 minutes, when the cauliflower is tender. Puree mixture until smooth (this will require you to blend a little at a time) and then return to soup pot. Add in milk and, stirring regularly, warm the soup. Season to taste with salt, pepper, parsley, and chili pepper. Serve with cashews and enjoy!

Dinner

You've done great all day so don't give up now! Your energy is high, you're feeling great, you've topped out on your workout and now you're ready to sit down to something delicious and filling. Dinner is typically the meal that those new to the vegan world begin to fear because it is the meal most commonly related to animal products. So how do we create meals and work around keeping meat off of our plates and out of our diets? You will be surprised at just how easy it is, and just how delicious these meals can be. There are many entrees here but there are also several side dishes that could be paired together for something new and interesting.

Chinese Sweet Potatoes

Ingredients

4 large sweet potatoes, cubed
2 tbsp olive oil
1 tsp kosher salt

¾ tbsp. Chinese five-spice powder
½ black pepper
3/-4 tbsp chopped chives

Directions

Preheat ove to 425F. On a baking sheet, toss sweet potatoes, oil, salt, pepper and spice. When coated, distribute evenly across baking sheet. Roast for 25 minutes or until tender. Sprinkle chives over top and serve.

Black Bean Burger

Ingredients:

3 cans black beans
12 oz chopped mushroom (Portobello)
2 chopped yellow onions
1 chopped green pepper
2 tbsp vegan Worcestershire
1 tbsp chili powder
½ tbsp. garlic powder
Paprika
Pinch of smoke flavor extract
1 tsp kosher salt
Black pepper
Whole wheat bread crumbs

Directions:

Sauté mushrooms, onions and peppers each separately until caramelized. Mash black beans and then add together all ingredients and mix well. Spray a large pan with non-stick spray. Heat pan on medium high. Cook burgers until browned on each side. Serve on whole wheat buns and top with some of your favorite veggies such as cucumber and spinach.

Broccoli Tofu Stir-Fry

Ingredients

12 oz firm tofu, cut into ½" thick cubes
1/3 cup + 1 tbsp tamari
1 ½ tbsp. rice wine vinegar (red wine vinegar can be substituted)
1/3 cup water
3 ½ tbsp maple syrup or agave nectar
1 ½ tbsp. lemon juice
1 ½ tsp toasted sesame oil
1 tsp blackstrap molasses
2 ½ tsp grated ginger
6 medium sized minced cloves of garlic
1 tbsp arrowroot powder
1 tbsp olive oil
5 cups broccoli cut into flowerets
1 tsp sea salt
2 tsp water
1 ½ cups sliced bell pepper (red, yellow, or orange)
1 tbsp teriyaki
¾ cup raw cashews
½ cup sliced green onion

Directions

Marinate tofu cubes by placing in shallow dish and pouring tamari and vinegar over them. Toss tofu to coat and evenly distribute. In a separate bowl, combine 1/3 cup water, syrup, lemon juice, sesame oil, molasses, ginger, garlic and arrowroot. Over high heat, sauté tofu in large sauce pan for 8 minutes, turning to evenly brown each side. Add broccoli and a pinch of salt and 2 tsp of water. Toss and cover for 2-3 minutes. As it turns to a brighter green, remove cover and add peppers. Sauté for another minute or two. Add teriyaki and increase to high heat. Toss to cover vegetables thoroughly. Allow sauce to come to slow boil and thicken before adding tofu, cashews and onions. Toss and remove from heat. Serve over noodles, rice, or quinoa.

*Optional: Add in other vegetables for added color and flavor, such as snow peas, zucchini, or carrots.

Roasted Potato Bowl *yields 3 servings*

Ingredients

6 cups, loosely packed, finely chopped collard greens with stems removed
4 tsp extra virgin olive oil
1 tsp apple cider vinegar
2 cloves garlic
1 tsp of salt
1 tsp of pepper
1 can chickpeas
Pinch of paprika, turmeric, cayenne, garlic powder
4 cups diced tiny red potatoes
2 tbsp extra virgin olive oil
2 tsp lemon juice
1/2 tsp garlic powder
1/8 tsp smoky paprika and/or cayenne
1 1/4 cups carrots
3 tbsp non-dairy milk
1 tbsp lemon juice
2 tbsp maple syrup
1/4 tsp freshly grated ginger

Pinch of orange zest
1 Satsuma orange, peeled and thinly sliced

Directions

Preheat oven to 420F. Add potatoes to large mixing bowl and toss with olive oil, lemon juice, pinch of salt and pepper. Spread onto baking sheet and bake until tender and crispy. About 5 minutes before they are done, sprinkle with garlic powder and paprika. Toss and continue baking. Drain and rinse chickpeas and toss with pinches of turmeric, paprika, cayenne and olive oil. Roast on baking sheet until edges crisp (about 10 minutes). While potatoes and chickpeas roast, boil a large pot of water and cook carrots until tender. Drain water and place in food processor. Add in milk, lemon juice, syrup, ginger, orange zest, a pinch of salt and pepper, and a pinch of cayenne. Blend to create dressing. Add a small amount of oil and garlic to a pot over high heat. Add in collards and cover. Cook for one minute, remove from heat, and toss. Pour in vinegar and a pinch of pepper. Toss. Add collards to bowl, top with sliced oranges, chickpeas, potatoes, and dressing.

Sweet Potato Bean Chili

Ingredients

2 tbsp extra virgin olive oil
1 large peeled and diced sweet potato
1 large diced red onion
4 cloves of minced garlic
2 tbsp chili powder
½ tsp ground chipotle pepper
½ tsp ground cumin
¼ tsp salt
3 ½ cups vegetable stock
1 can black beans, rinsed
1 can diced tomatoes
½ cup dried quinoa
4 tsp lime juice

Directions

Heat oil in large sauce pan over medium high heat. Add sweet potato and onion, cooking until onion becomes soft. Stir in garlic, chili powder, chipotle, cumin and salt. Stir in stock, tomatoes, black beans and quinoa and bring to boil. Continue stirring. Cover and reduce heat to medium low and simmer for 10 minutes or until quinoa is cooked and potatoes are soft. Add lime juice and remove from heat. Season with salt.

*Optional: Garnish with avocado, cilantro, or cream cheese before serving.

Veggie and Chimichurri Hash *yields 3*

servings

Ingredients

3 small white sweet potatoes, chopped
1 large bunch of asparagus
5 medium green onions
2 tbsp coconut oil
1 cup parsley, finely chopped
1 ½ full cups of cilantro, finely chopped
3 cloves of crushed garlic
5 tbsp finely minced shallot

2 tbsp fresh lemon juice
1 1/2 cups olive oil
1/4 cup red wine vinegar
Pinch of salt and pepper

Directions

Stir together olive oil, vinegar, lemon juice, parley, cilantro, garlic, shallots and ¾ tsp salt to create chimichurri sauce. Allow to sit while preparing the rest of the meal to allow the flavors to develop. Boil large pot of salted water. Slice green onions into thin rounds. Chop asparagus into 1" pieces. Cook potatoes in boiling water until fork tender, but not too soft. Add asparagus and cook 2 more minutes. Sauté green onion in coconut oil over medium low heat. Add a pinch of salt. Drain sweet potatoes and combine with green onions adding a small amount of coconut oil and a pinch of salt and pepper. Sauté over medium heat, turning every few minutes to allow time to brown evenly. Add another small amount of coconut oil if they begin to stick or dry out. Serve with chimichurri sauce mixture poured over.

Lemon Garlic Brussel Sprouts

Ingredients

2 lbs trimmed and halved Brussel sprouts
3 tbsp Olive Oil
1 tbsp Butter
1 tsp Red Pepper Flakes
4 cloves chopped garlic
1 Lemon, zested and juiced

Directions

Heat olive oil over medium high heat in large skillet. Add Brussel sprouts and sauté until light brown and fork tender. Add butter, red pepper and garlic and sauté for 1 minute. Remove from heat and stir in remaining ingredients.

Sweet Potato Patties *yields 12 patties*

Ingredients:

2 medium sweet potatoes, cooked and mashed (about 2 cups worth)
2 cups cooked quinoa
1 medium yellow onion, diced
3 cloves of crushed garlic
1 tbsp finely chopped fresh thyme
1 tbsp extra virgin olive oil
Pinch of sea salt
Pinch of black pepper
Coconut oil

Directions:

In a saucepan over medium low heat, sauté onions, olive oil and sea salt until onions are translucent. Add garlic and cook one minute, stirring constantly to prevent burning. Add thyme and stir. Add onions, quinoa, ¼ tsp sea salt, pepper, and sweet potatoes and stir until mixed well. Form small, golf ball sized balls from mixture and then flatten into patties. In nonstick pan, add small amount of coconut oil and fry patties 2 minutes per side (or until brown and crisp). Top with thyme leave and a sprinkle of salt and serve.

Cheesy Acorn Alfredo

1 medium acorn squash, roasted
1 cup parsley
3/4 cup almond or soy milk
1/3 cup yeast flakes
3 Tbsp extra virgin olive oil
3 Tbsp Dijon Mustard
3 Tbsp apple cider vinegar
2 Tbsp roasted garlic
2 Tbsp dried Italian herbs mixture
1 Tbsp maple syrup
1 tsp red pepper flakes
salt and pepper
1 bag pasta (any variety you'd like)
3 cups mushrooms
1 package cubed tempeh
1 tube chipotle vegan sausage
1 tbsp Daiya Cheese on top

Directions:

Preheat oven to 300F. Bring a large pot of salter water to a boil and cook pasta. When pasta is nearly done (about 3 minutes left), add in mushrooms, sausage and tempeh. Drain when cooked fully. Add remaining ingredients to blender or food processor until well blended (about 2 minutes). Toss pasta and sauce until pasta is well coated. Transfer to casserole dish and bake for 20 minutes. Sprinkle with daiya cheese and serve.

Lentil Burgers yield 8 small burgers

Ingredients

1 small onion, chopped
1/2 cup dry short-grain brown rice
1/2 cup dry lentils
3/4 teaspoon salt
2 cups water

1 medium, finely chopped celery stalk
1 small carrot, finely chopped
2 tsp stone-ground mustard
1 tsp garlic powder
Vegetable oil spray

Directions

Stir together water, salt, rice, lentils, and onion in medium saucepan and bring to a simmer. Cover and cook for about 50 minutes or until rice is tender and water is absorbed. Add carrots, celery, mustard, and garlic powder to mixture, stirring well, and then chill for several hours to allow for easier patty forming. Once cooled, mold mixture into small patties, about 3 inches in diameter. Spray nonstick skillet and cook patties over medium high heat until lightly browned on each side.

Snacks and Desserts

Do you have a sugar addiction? Even those most disciplined with their diets tend to struggle most when it comes to sugar, specifically with their snack foods. Is it possible to have healthy, energy inducing, fat burning, heart healthy snacks and still satisfy that sweet tooth? Being health conscious should never mean that you can't give into your cravings. The trick is moderation and understanding what we are putting in our food. Of course it's easier to go buy a bag of potato chips, a box of cookies, or a carton of ice cream, but once you've indulged, you lean back on the couch, and realize that you feel a little bit of misery for every single bite you took, will you still feel that it was worth it? What about diving into your desires, and still feeling amazing at the end of the day? With these recipes, not only will you know exactly what you are eating, but you'll also feel better about it, too.

Apple Pie and Whipped Cream

Yields 10-12 pies

Ingredients:

6 large peeled and sliced apples
1 1/3 cups water
1 1/4 tbsp lemon juice
1 cup + 1 tsp sugar
3 tbsp cornstarch
4 pinches of sea salt
2 tsp cinnamon
1 tsp nutmeg
24 spring roll wrappers, defrosted on counter for an hour before use (it may be difficult to find vegan friendly versions, so you may have to order them online)
Non-stick spray
3 Tablespoons melted vegan butter
1/4 cup Cinnamon sugar mix
2 cans of full-fat coconut milk, unshaken and chilled
3 tsp vanilla

Directions:

To make whipped topping, open coconut milk and scrape out only the solid white portion from the top of the first can, leaving the liquid into a bowl. Shake second can and add entirety of contents to bowl. Add in vanilla and 1 tsp of sugar, beating with mixer until fluffy. Refrigerate. Over medium heat, mix apples, water, lemon juice, 1 cup of sugar, cornstarch and salt in a saucepan. When it begins to simmer, reduce to medium low and cook until apples soften (about 25 minutes), stirring regularly. Add more water, if needed. Spring roll wrappers can be tricky, so take your time when peeling them apart. Use water to keep them moist while separating them (you can pull two apart at a time, as they will need to be doubled up for the recipe). When apple filling is ready is ready, place wrappers (two ply thick) on nonstick surface like a diamond and spoon two spoonful's into center. Take the top of the diamond and fold it down to meet the bottom. Take each side point and fold them in towards one another and then take the bottom point and fold it up and around the roll. Heat the grill to medium low heat and spray with nonstick spray.

Grill rolls, folded sides facing down for about 5 minutes. Flip and grill for another 5 minutes. Be careful not to burn them and only to get grill marks. Brush over with butter and sprinkle with cinnamon sugar mixture. Serve with coconut whipped cream on top!

Cranberry and Seed Granola Bars *yields 10-12 bars*

Ingredients

¾ cup oat flour
1 cup water
¾ cup packed pitted dates
½ cup chia seeds
½ cup uncooked sunflower seeds
½ cup uncooked pumpkin seeds
½ cup finely chopped, dried cranberries
1 teaspoon cinnamon
1 teaspoon vanilla extract
½ tsp fine grain sea salt

Optional Additives: Sliced Almonds, 1 tbsp coconut oil, peanut butter, and anything else you can imagine!

Directions

Preheat oven to 325F and line a small cookie sheet or 9x9 pan with parchment paper. Combine water and dates and allow to soak for up to 30 minutes if they are firm. Blend until they are smooth. Combine all ingredients into large bowl until well blended. Using a spatula or slightly damp hands, spread mixture evenly into pan, pressing lightly into the dish so the granola bars will be firm. Bake for 20-25 minutes or until firm. Allow to cook for 5 minutes and then using parchment, pull from pan and allow to cook on cooling rack.

*Unlike store bought granola bars, these do not last indefinitely. Seal tightly at room temperature for up to a week or freeze any leftovers.

Citrus Granola Parfait *yields 4 servings*

Ingredients:

Zest of 1/2 lemon
Zest of 1/2 lime
Zest of 1/2 orange
1 1/2 tbsp grape seed oil
2 tbsp orange juice
2 tbsp lemon juice
1 tbsp lime juice
1 1/2 tbsp maple syrup
1/2 tsp vanilla extract
1 cup rolled oats
1/8 cup pumpkin seeds
1/8 cup sunflower seeds
1/8 cup raw walnuts, chopped
1/8 cup almonds, chopped
1/8 cup unsweetened dried coconut
1/8 cup flax seed
1/8 cup dried apricots, chopped

1/8 cup dried cranberries
16 ounces vanilla soy yogurt

Preheat your oven to 300F. Mix together all ingredients except yogurt and spread into large pan or cookie sheet. Bake for 15 minutes, stir, and bake for another 15 minutes. Remove from oven and cool for 10 minutes. To serve, alternate granola and scoops of yogurt.

*Optional: Mix in fruit when serving with yogurt, such as chopped strawberries, blueberries, chopped mango, or even pineapple bits.

Potato Pudding yields 3 servings

Ingredients

1/3 cup rolled oats
1/2 cup fortified soy or rice milk
1 cup cooked sweet potato or yam
1 tablespoon maple syrup
1/4 teaspoon cinnamon

Directions

Combine all ingredients in a blender and blend until smooth. Serve warm or allow to chill before serving!

Conclusion

It is just as important to feed your body as it is to strengthen it, but you don't have to give up on wonderful foods or eat foods that compromise your health in order to do it. It's a great idea to incorporate a variety of raw foods into your diet, but sometimes that just isn't enough. We crave flavors, sometimes we crave the sweets, and to not give into those cravings can result in failure. So give in, add a little texture and excitement to your pallet and enjoy the fact that you are giving your body exactly what it's asking for! Stay hydrated, stay active, stay healthy!

Part 2

Introduction

Yes, dessert! Everyone's favorite part of the meal.

For ages, people have been tossing dairy and eggs into desserts wily-nilly, with no thought of how it affects us poor vegans.

But those days are changing. People are discovering that you don't need animal products to make delicious and crowd-pleasing desserts.

The following recipes are designed to give you a broad range of recipes so you can create typical desserts that will hit your sweet spot, while keeping strictly vegan.

We have recipes spanning all types of cookies, cakes, brownies, and even non-dairy ice creams.

I sincerely hope you find something in there that you and your family will enjoy.

A quick note: when looking for many of these ingredients, specifically chocolate chips or powder, margarine, shortening and sugar, be aware that many companies add animal products to these ingredients. So be sure to carefully read the ingredients list before purchasing any of these ingredients.

With that said, let's get to the recipes!

Fudge Brownies

Let's start this book off right - with some decadent, you'd-never-believe-they-were-vegan brownies. For bonus points, serve these with one of the following ice cream recipes.

Ingredients

6 Tbsp water
2 Tbsp golden flax meal
1 3/4 cups all-purpose flour
1/4 tsp baking soda
7 Tbsp cocoa powder
4 ounces semi-sweet chocolate, chopped into 1/4 inch pieces
1 tsp instant espresso powder
3/4 tsp salt
1/4 cup boiling water
1 1/2 cups sugar
6 Tbsp stick margarine
1 1/2 tsp vanilla extract

Instructions

Preheat your oven to 350 degrees.

Prepare your "flax eggs": in a small bowl or mug, whisk together the 6 Tbsp water with the 2 Tbsp flax meal, and let sit for about 10 minutes. Set aside.

Line an 8-inch by 8-inch baking dish with parchment paper. Let some excess paper hang over the sides. This will make it easy to remove the brownies from the hot dish after baking.

In another bowl, whisk together the flour and baking soda, and set aside.

In yet another bowl, combine the cocoa powder, semi-sweet chocolate, espresso powder and salt. Add in 1/4 cup of boiling water, and use a wooden spoon to mix everything together until the chocolate is all melted.

Now add in the sugar, margarine, vanilla extract and the flax "egg" mixture. Using an electric hand mixer, mix until smooth.

Now add in the flour/baking soda mixture. Use your hands to mix the ingredients until just combined, but don't over-mix at this point.

Transfer this batter to the parchment-lined baking dish, spread the batter evenly in the dish and bake for about 25 minutes.

Upon removal from the oven, remove the brownies from the dish by grabbing the sides of the parchment paper and lifting. Let the brownies cool for about an hour (on a wire rack if you have one), and then cut into squares.

Vanilla Ice Cream

With this and the next few recipes, we will be exploring variations of dairy-free ice cream made with coconut milk. Feel free to experiment with additional flavors, but these are some of my favorites. If you have an ice cream machine, feel free to use it, but I have included instructions for the less-prepared ice cream fans among us.

For this recipe, I firmly believe you can't go wrong with the deceptively complex flavor of vanilla ice cream.

Ingredients

One 13.5-ounce can of full-fat coconut milk, placed overnight in the fridge

1 cup almond milk

2 Tbsp vanilla extract
3 Tbsp white sugar
1/4 tsp table salt

Instructions

Pop open the can of coconut milk and scoop out the top, solid layer into a mixing bowl. Discard the leftover coconut water, or drink, or use in a different recipe.

Add in the almond milk, vanilla extract, sugar and salt. Whisk everything together vigorously until the sugar is dissolved.

Put the bowl in the freezer. Take out and whisk every half hour until frozen (total time 3-4 hours).

This recipe keeps in the freezer for about a week. Remove from the freezer about 5-10 minutes before serving.

Choco Peanut Butter Ice Cream

This recipe combines two of my favorite things - chocolate and peanut butter - into a creamy frozen treat.

Ingredients

2 large frozen bananas - sliced
2 Tbsp cocoa powder
2 Tbsp creamy peanut butter

1/2 tsp vanilla
1/4 tsp cinnamon
Pinch of salt
Instructions
Combine all the ingredients in a blender or food processor. Blend/process for 15 seconds at a time, until the mixture is smooth and creamy.

Serve immediately, or place in the freezer for later.

Mint Chocolate Chip Ice Cream

This is a good one for the guests. The spinach we are using is just for color, not flavor.

Ingredients

About 1/2 cup fresh baby spinach (We will just use this for color.)

3 13.5-ounce cans of full-fat coconut milk - chilled in the fridge overnight

3/4 cup honey or maple syrup

1 1/2 tbsp peppermint extract

1 cup chocolate chips

Instructions

Place spinach in a blender along with a few Tbsp of water. Blend until smooth and transfer to a saucepan. Cook over medium heat until the liquid has reduced. Remove from heat and set aside to cool.

Open the cans of coconut milk and scoop out the fatty solid layers, discarding or using the coconut water in another recipe.

In a bowl, combine 1 Tbsp of the spinach puree with a little bit of the coconut milk, whisking together until fully combined and smooth. (We are only using this 1 Tbsp of the spinach puree, as it is just for the green color.)

Add in the rest of the ingredients (but no more spinach puree!), and whip together until everything is smooth and creamy.

(Optional) Add the chocolate chips to a food processor or blender and pulse once, just to break up the chips a bit.

Put in the freezer to chill, removing to whisk vigorously every half hour. It should be frozen in 3-4 hours.

Maple Walnut Ice Cream

Another tasty ice cream recipe, this time with a maple syrup kick.

Ingredients

4 cups water

16 ounces of coconut butter

1 1/2 cup maple syrup
2 tsp Celtic Sea salt
1 cup walnuts (soaked for an hour, drained and roughly chopped)

Instructions

In a blender, combine water, coconut butter, maple syrup and salt. Blend until smooth and place in a bowl in the freezer for 3-4 hours, removing every half hour to whisk vigorously. Add in the walnuts as the ice cream firms up.

Salted Bourbon Caramel Ice Cream

Need more booze flavor in your dessert? This recipe has it, plus the bourbon creates some nice layers of flavor complexity.

Ingredients

1 1/2 cups raw cashews, soaked for a couple hours, then drained
1 cup bourbon
1/2 cup organic cane sugar
4 Tbsp unsweetened almond milk
1/4 tsp salt
1 13.5-ounce can of full fat coconut milk
3 Tbsp coconut oil, melted
1 tsp vanilla extract
1/4 cup agave nectar

Instructions

In a small saucepan over medium heat, bring the bourbon and sugar to a boil. Reduce heat to low to simmer, and swirl the liquid until a caramel forms. Make sure to keep a close eye, since it tends to happen all at once.

After the caramel forms, remove from heat and immediately add in 3 Tbsp of almond milk and the salt, and stir. Set aside to cool.

Add the remaining almond milk, cashews, coconut milk, coconut oil, vanilla extract and agave nectar to a blender. Blend until smooth and creamy, scraping the sides with a spatula as needed. It may take a couple of minutes for the cashews to completely liquify.

Add half of the bourbon caramel mixture and blend again.

Chill the remaining half of the bourbon caramel in the fridge.

Place in the freezer for 3-4 hours, removing every half hour to whisk vigorously. When almost frozen solid, stir in the remaining bourbon caramel to give a marbled effect.

Let thaw for 5-10 minutes before serving the ice cream.

Chocolate Chip Cookies

Another staple of the vegan kitchen. Seriously, why would you bake non-vegan cookies?

Ingredients

2 1/2 cups all-purpose flour

1 tsp baking soda

1 tsp fine salt

2 sticks (8 ounces) unsalted margarine, at room temperature

1 1/4 cups granulated sugar

1 Tbsp light molasses

2 tsp vanilla extract

1 1/2 cups vegan semisweet chocolate chips

Instructions

Preheat the oven to 350 degrees.

In a mixing bowl, combine flour, baking soda and salt and whisk together until combined.

In a mixing bowl (or stand mixer), place the margarine and sugar. Mix well with a hand mixer (or your stand mixer) until the mixture is light and fluffy. Add in the molasses and vanilla extract and mix again.

Add in the flour mixture and mix on the low setting until just combined (do not over-mix at this point). Add in the chocolate chips and mix until just combined.

Onto a dry (un-greased) baking sheet, drop the dough 1 heaping Tbsp at a time. Roll the ball and press down on the top to slightly flatten. Space out the balls about 2 inches from each other.

Bake one sheet at a time, about 10-12 minutes until the cookies are lightly golden at the edges. Remove and cool on the baking sheet for a few minutes. Then remove and allow to cool completely on a wire rack (if you have one).

Repeat the baking process until you are out of cookie dough. Make sure to use a cool baking sheet with each batch.

Peanut Butter Cookies

I thoroughly enjoy a soft peanut butter cookie. The cross-hatch pattern on top of the cookies makes it look like you really know what you're doing!

Ingredients

1 cup peanut butter

1 cup brown sugar

2 tsp vanilla extract

2/3 cup oat flour

1 tsp baking soda

1/8 tsp salt

1/4 cup water

Instructions

Preheat oven to 350 degrees and line two baking sheets with parchment paper.

In a mixing bowl, mix together the peanut butter and brown sugar using a hand mixer. Add in the vanilla extract and mix again until combined.

In another mixing bowl, mix together the oat flour, baking soda and salt until well-combined.

Now, combine the two mixtures: while beating the peanut butter-sugar mixture with a hand mixer, slowly add in the oat flour mixture until a dough starts to form. Add in water and beat until well-mixed. Make sure not to over-mix at this point.

Form balls of dough using about 1 1/2 – 2 Tbsp of dough per cookie and drop onto the parchment paper. Flatten with a fork one way, then the other way, to create a criss-cross pattern on the top of each ball.

Bake for 8-10 minutes until cookies are just barely golden at the edges.

Let cool on the baking sheet for a few minutes, then remove to cool on a wire rack and serve.

Dark Chocolate Macaroons

A nice little coconut-based cookie, with an optional dark chocolate bottom. I know you will like these - just make sure your guests or loved ones don't hate coconut.

Ingredients

3 cups shredded unsweetened coconut
1/4 tsp vanilla extract
2 Tbsp maple syrup
1/2 Tbsp melted coconut oil
1/2 cup dark chocolate, chopped (optional)

Instructions

Preheat oven to 350 degrees and line a baking sheet with parchment paper.

Add coconut to a blender or food processor and blend/process until the coconut is almost buttery, but not too liquid-y.

Add in the maple syrup and vanilla extract and blend/process until just combined.

Using between 1-1 1/2 Tbsp per cookie, use your hands to pack together a tight ball and drop onto the parchment paper. Gently press down to flatten the macaroon into a half-sphere. Brush the top with melted coconut oil and sprinkle with any leftover coconut crumbs.

Bake for 8-10 minutes, until the edges are just slightly brown. Remove from oven and set aside.

(Optional) Melt the dark chocolate using a double broiler (or using the microwave in short increments). Once the macaroons are cooled, pick one up and dip the bottom in the melted chocolate. Place on a parchment-lined plate until the chocolate has set.

Serve.

Snickerdoodles

Just the word "snickerdoodle" takes me back to my childhood, to a warm and cozy kitchen looking out on a snowy back yard. Sigh.

Ingredients

For the cookie dough

1 3/4 cup all-purpose flour

1/4 cup cornstarch

1 tsp. baking powder

1 stick (4 oz.) vegan margarine, at room temperature

3/4 cup sugar

1/4 cup vanilla almond milk

1 tsp vanilla extract

Cinnamon sugar

1/2 cup sugar

3 Tbsp ground cinnamon

Instructions

Preheat oven to 350 degrees and coat a baking sheet with cooking spray (or cover with parchment paper).

Make the cookie dough

In a mixing bowl, whisk together the flour, cornstarch and baking powder. In a separate bowl, use hand mixer to beat together the margarine and sugar until light and fluffy. Mix in the almond milk and vanilla extract and beat another 30 seconds until smooth and well-mixed. Add in the flour mixture and beat 30 seconds, until smooth but not overly mixed.

Make the cinnamon sugar

Combine cinnamon and sugar on a plate.

Shape the dough into 1-inch balls. Roll each ball in the cinnamon sugar and drop onto the baking sheet, spaced 2 inches apart.

Bake for 10-12 minutes, until golden at the edges.

Remove from oven, and let cool 5 minutes on the baking sheet. Then remove to a wire rack and let cool completely.

Gingerbread Cookies

It just ain't the holidays without some gingerbread cookies. Get some colored icing and decorate these for a fun family activity!

Ingredients

1 1/3 cups whole wheat flour

3/4 cup all purpose flour

1/2 Tbsp baking powder

1 tsp baking soda

1/2 Tbsp cinnamon

2 tsp ginger

1/2 tsp nutmeg

1/2 tsp cloves

1/2 cup coconut oil

1/2 cup + 1 Tbsp sugar

1/4 cup water

1/2 cup molasses

1/2 tsp vanilla extract

Instructions

Preheat oven to 325 degrees.

In a mixing bowl, combine the flours, baking powder, baking soda, cinnamon, ginger, nutmeg and cloves.

In a different bowl, mix together the coconut oil and sugar using a hand mixer. Beat until the mixture is light and fluffy. Add in the water, vanilla extract and molasses, and beat another 30 seconds until just combined. Slowly add in the flour mixture while beating, until just combined. Wrap the dough in plastic wrap and place in the fridge for at least two hours.

On removing from the fridge, let the dough sit for at least a half hour until it is room temperature.

Roll the dough onto parchment paper until the dough is about 1/4-inch thick.

Use cookie cutters to cut the dough, until the dough is all used.

Place the unbaked cookies in the freezer for 10 minutes to harden a bit.

Remove cookies from the freezer and place on a parchment-lined baking sheet.

Bake for 8-10 minutes, until the cookies are golden at the edges.

Remove from oven and let cool on a wire rack.

Decorate however you like, or just serve as is!

Shortbread Cookies

Some simple shortbread cookies. Great for dunking in your tea, especially if you are prone to calling these "biscuits."

Ingredients

1/2 cup margarine, at room temperature

1/3 cup maple syrup

2 1/4 cups all-purpose flour

1/4 tsp vanilla extract

Dash of salt

Instructions

Preheat your oven to 350 degrees and line a baking sheet with parchment paper.

Place margarine in a large mixing bowl and beat with a hand mixer until creamy.

Add in the maple syrup, salt and vanilla extract and mix again until well-combined.

Slowly add in your flour while stirring with a spoon, then knead with your hands until you can form it into a doughy ball.

Take your dough and roll it into a 1/2-inch thick disc or rectangle. Use a cookie or pizza cutter to cut out 1-inch by 3-inch rectangles. Place each rectangle on the prepared baking sheet and poke a few holes in the top with a fork to avoid cracking.

Bake for 15 minutes, until the edges are lightly golden. Remove from oven and cool on a wire rack.

Chewy Molasses Cookies

Sweet and chewy, what more do you want from a cookie?

Ingredients

1 cup all-purpose flour
3/4 tsp baking soda

1/2 tsp baking powder
1/2 tsp cinnamon
1/4 tsp nutmeg
1/4 tsp salt
1/4 cup vegan margarine
1/2 cup sugar
2 tbsp canola oil
2 tbsp molasses
1/4 cup sugar for rolling

Instructions

Preheat your oven to 350 degrees. Line a baking sheet with parchment paper.

In a small bowl combine flour, baking soda, baking powder, cinnamon, nutmeg and salt. Whisk until well-combined.

In a large mixing bowl, use a hand mixer to beat together the margarine and 1/2 cup sugar until the mixture is nice and fluffy. Add in the oil and molasses and mix again until well-combined.

Start to slowly add in the dry flour mixture while you stir with a wooden spoon. Mix until just combined. Don't over-mix at this point.

Place the 1/4 cup sugar on a plate or in a small bowl. Take about 1 Tbsp of dough and roll into a ball. Coat the dough in the sugar and place on your prepared baking sheet. Repeat with the rest of the dough.

Bake for 10-12 minutes, or until the edges start to brown. Remove from oven and allow to cool on the sheet for a few minutes, then remove to a wire rack to cool completely.

Chocolate-Covered Frozen Banana Bites

This is a tasty treat that will impress your guests - frozen banana slices with a thick chocolate shell.

Ingredients

2 medium ripe bananas, sliced into 1/2-inch rounds

1/2 cup dark chocolate chips

1 Tbsp coconut oil

*Optional add ins/ons – chopped nuts, shredded coconut, peanut or almond butter

Instructions

Place the bananas on a parchment-lined baking sheet and pop in the freer for about 2 hours.

When the bananas are frozen, melt together the chocolate and coconut oil in a small saucepan over low heat.

Remove the bananas from the freezer and use a fork or toothpick to dip each banana slice in the melted chocolate. Shake off any excess and place back on the parchment-lined sheet.

Serve immediately or put the sheet back in the freezer for later.

Peanut Butter Chocolate Balls

This recipe has a bunch of steps, but it's not too complex. Just take it slow. First, you make the caramel and mix with the peanut butter, roll into balls, then melt the chocolate and cover the balls with it. Then add the peanut butter crumbs.

Ingredients

1/2 cup sugar

3 Tbsp water

1 Tbsp margarine

1/3 tsp salt

1/2 cup smooth, unsalted peanut butter

1/4 cup peanuts, processed into small bits

7 ounces semi-sweet chocolate

Instructions

First, set up your ice water bath. This is a mixing bowl filled with ice water that is larger than the small saucepan you will use to make the caramel mixture.

Next, add the sugar, water, margarine and salt to your small saucepan over medium-low heat. Stir occasionally until your sugar thermometer reads 230 degrees. Now dunk the saucepan into your ice water bath so that the mixture stops cooking. Whisk in the peanut butter until smooth and well-combined. Transfer to a bowl and set in the freezer for 15 minutes to cool off a bit.

Remove the peanut butter mixture from the freezer and knead on a flat surface. Form into one-inch balls in your hand, place on a parchment-lined cookie sheet and put back in the freezer to chill for an hour.

Using a double boiler, melt the semi-sweet chocolate until completely liquified and then turn off the heat.

Get your peanut butter balls out of the freezer. Roll each ball in the melted chocolate, place back on the baking sheet and sprinkle with the ground peanuts. When finished with all the balls, place the sheet back in the fewer for another hour so that the chocolate can set.

Dark Chocolate Truffles

I never thought I could make these myself. But they're not that difficult!

Ingredients

8 ounces dark chocolate, chopped

1/4 cup unrefined coconut oil

3 Tbsp water

1 tsp vanilla extract

Pinch of salt

1/4 cup unsweetened cocoa powder

Optional toppings: cocoa powder, finely chopped peanuts, shredded coconut

Instructions

Melt chocolate in a double boiler with the oil and the water. Remove from heat and stir in the vanilla extract and salt. Transfer to an 8-inch square baking dish, and chill in the fridge for two hours.

Using a melon baller (if you have one), make one-inch chocolate balls and place on a parchment-lined baking sheet. Chill the entire baking sheet for about ten minutes.

Remove from fridge, add optional toppings and serve.

Cinnamon Rolls

These taste just like the rolls you find at Cinnabon, but you actually know what goes into these, which is a plus.

Ingredients

Dough

1 cup almond milk, warmed

1 0.75-ounce packet of dry active yeast

1/3 cup margarine

1/2 cup granulated sugar

Dash of salt

4 1/2 cups of all purpose flour

Filling

1 cup brown sugar

2 Tbsp cinnamon

1/3 cup margarine

Icing

1 8-ounce package vegan cream cheese

1/4 cup nondairy margarine

2 cups confectioner's sugar

1 tsp vanilla

2 Tbsp water

Instructions

Make the dough

Mix the yeast with the warm almond milk, and let the mixture rest for about 5 minutes, until it appears frothy. Using a hand mixer or strong whisk, mix in the 1/3 cup margarine, 1/2 cup of sugar and the dash of salt until everything is smooth and well-combined. As you continue mixing, gradually add in the flour. You will have to abandon the hand mixer and use your hands. Knead the dough for about 7-8 minutes, then place in a lightly greased bowl in a warm part of your kitchen for an hour to rise.

After the dough has risen, roll onto a lightly floured surface or parchment paper. We are aiming for about 16-inch by 20-inch rectangle of dough.

Preheat the oven to 400 degrees.

Make the filling

Using a hand mixer, mix together the brown sugar, cinnamon and 1/3 cup margarine until light and fluffy.

Spread this mixture evenly over your dough rectangle.

Now, tightly roll the rectangle from the long side, so that the resulting dough cylinder is still 20-inches long.

Cut the cylinder into 12 equally sized rolls, and place the rolls in a baking pan, covered loosely with a kitchen towel. Allow the rolls to rise for 30 minutes.

Now place the pan in the oven (minus the towel) and bake for 15-20 minutes, until the rolls are golden brown at the edges.

Make the icing

While the rolls are in the oven, use a hand mixer or strong whisk to combine the vegan cream cheese, confectioner's sugar, vanilla extract and water until the mixture is light and fluffy. We are looking for a thick sauce-like texture.

Finish the job

Remove the rolls from the oven and immediately invert the rolls into a different pan, to allow the cinnamon-sugar to re-coat the rolls. Let cool for ten minutes and slather icing on top of the rolls.

Serve warm or at room temperature.

Vanilla Cupcakes

Vanilla-on-vanilla cupcakes are my personal favorite, and the yardstick I use to judge any new cupcake shop I visit.

Ingredients

For the cake

1 1/4 cups all-purpose flour

1/2 cup plus 1/3 cup white sugar

1 tsp baking soda

1/2 tsp salt

2/3 cup unsweetened almond milk

1/3 cup canola oil

2 Tbsp apple cider vinegar

2 tsp vanilla extract

For the icing

1/4 cup vegan shortening

1/4 cup margarine

1 1/2 cups powdered sugar

1/2 tsp vanilla extract

2 Tbsp unsweetened almond milk

Sprinkles (optional)

Instructions

Make the cake

Preheat the oven to 350 degrees.

Grease your cupcake pan, or line with 12 paper cupcake liners.

In a mixing bowl, whisk together the dry cake ingredients (flour, sugar, baking soda, salt) until well-combined.

In a separate mixing bowl, combine the wet cake ingredients (almond milk, oil, vinegar, vanilla extract).

Now pour the wet ingredients into the bowl of dry ingredients and whisk until just-combined (don't over mix at this point).

Pour the batter evenly into the 12 liners and pop the pan into the oven.

Bake for 18-20 minutes, until the tops are lightly golden. Remove from the oven and set aside to cool.

Make the icing

Add the frosting ingredients to a mixing bowl (shortening, margarine, powdered sugar, vanilla extract, almond milk), and mix with a hand mixer until the icing is fluffy.

When the cupcakes are cool, spread the icing on the cupcakes and serve.

Red Velvet Cupcakes with Cream Cheese Frosting

Yes, the red just comes from food coloring. But the real star of this recipe is the "cream cheese" frosting.

Ingredients

For the cake

1 cup soy milk

1 tsp apple cider vinegar

1 1/4 cups all-purpose flour

1 cup granulated sugar

2 Tbsp cocoa powder

1/2 tsp baking powder

1/2 tsp baking soda

1/2 tsp salt

1/3 cup canola oil

2 Tbsp red food coloring

2 tsp vanilla extract

1/4 tsp almond extract

1 tsp chocolate extract

For the frosting

1/4 cup margarine, at room temperature

1/4 cup vegan cream cheese, at room temperature

1 1/2 cups powdered sugar

1 tsp vanilla extract

Instructions

Make the cupcakes

Preheat oven to 350 degrees. Line your cupcake pan with paper cupcake liners or lightly grease the pan.

In a small bowl, mix together the soy milk and vinegar and set aside to curdle.

In a large bowl, combine the flour, cocoa powder, sugar, baking powder, baking soda and salt and mix until well-combined.

Once the soy milk has curdled, add oil, food coloring, chocolate extract, vanilla extract and almond extract to the small bowl and whisk to combine well.

Add the soy milk mixture to the bowl of dry ingredients and mix until the ingredients are just combined. Do not over-mix.

Now pour the batter into your paper liners or cupcake pan, filling only about 3/4 of each cupcake liner.

Bake for 18-20 minutes, until a toothpick inserted in the cake comes out clean.

Remove from oven and allow to cool for about an hour.

Make the frosting

In a bowl, combine margarine and vegan cream cheese and mix with a hand mixer until just combined. Slowly add in the powdered sugar while you continue to mix, until the mixture is smooth, creamy, and a bit fluffy. Mix in the vanilla extract.

When the cupcakes have completely cooled, spread icing on top and serve.

Chocolate Cake

Chocolate-on-chocolate cake is what dessert is all about. If it's too much chocolate for your taste, switch out the icing for another you find in this book!

Ingredients

For the cake

1 1/4 cups flour

1 cup sugar

1/3 cup unsweetened cocoa powder

1 tsp baking soda

1/2 tsp salt

1 cup warm water

1 tsp vanilla extract

1/3 cup vegetable oil

1 tsp white or apple cider vinegar

For the icing

1/2 cup sugar

4 Tbsp margarine

2 Tbsp almond milk

2 Tbsp unsweetened cocoa powder

2 tsp vanilla extract

Instructions

Make the cake

Preheat oven to 350 degrees.

In a mixing bowl, combine the flour, sugar, cocoa powder, baking soda and salt, and stir until well-combined. Now add in the water, vanilla extract, vegetable oil and vinegar, and whisk together until well-combined.

Pour the mixture into a 8-inch square baking dish, and bake for about 30 minutes, until a toothpick inserted in the center comes out clean.

Remove from the oven and allow to cool completely (at least an hour).

Make the icing

While the cake is cooling, combine in a small saucepan the sugar, margarine, almond milk and cocoa powder, and bring to a boil, stirring often. After bring to a boil, reduce the heat to a simmer, and stir constantly for 2 minutes. Remove from heat and continue to stir for another 5 minutes.

Add in the vanilla extract, and stir again. Spread the icing on top of the cake immediately, and allow to cool for about an hour before serving.

Cinnamon Coffee Cake

My grandfather used to eat this for breakfast. I don't recommend that, but this cake will go great with coffee after a dinner party.

Ingredients

For the cake

1 cup almond milk

1/3 cup canola oil

1 Tbsp white vinegar

1 cup all-purpose flour

1/2 cup granulated sugar

1 tsp baking powder

1 tsp baking soda

2 tsp ground cinnamon

1 tsp ground ginger

1/4 tsp salt

For the crumble

3/4 cup all-purpose flour

1/4 cup brown sugar

2 tsp ground cinnamon

1/2 tsp ground ginger

1/4 tsp salt
3/4 cup chopped walnuts
1/3 cup margarine, melted

Instructions

Preheat the oven to 350 degrees and lightly grease a 9-inch square baking dish.

Make the cake

In a large mixing bowl, combine the flour, sugar, baking powder, baking soda, cinnamon, ginger and salt, and whisk until well-combined.

In a separate bowl, combine the wet cake ingredients (almond milk, oil, vinegar) and stir until combined.

Now, add the wet ingredients to the bowl of dry ingredients and stir with a whisk or fork until just combined. Do not over mix at this point.

Pour the batter into the greased baking dish

Make the crumble

In a small bowl, combine the flour, sugar, cinnamon, ginger, salt and walnuts and whisk until well-combined.

Add in the melted margarine and work the mixture until al of the dry ingredients are coated.

Spoon the crumble mixture on top of the batter in the pan, covering the batter evenly.

Bake the cake

Bake for 35-40 minutes, until a toothpick or knife inserted in the cake comes out clean.

Let cool for a half hour and serve warm or at room temperature.

Pineapple Upside-Down Cake

This one is a throwback, but what's not to like about a pineapple upside-down cake? Plus, it's just fun to make.

Ingredients

1/2 cup vegan margarine

1/2 cup brown sugar

One can of pineapple slices

Maraschino cherries

2 1/2 cups all-purpose flour

1 1/3 cups sugar

2 tsp baking powder

1/2 tsp salt

1/2 cup canola oil

1 cup almond milk
1 tsp vanilla extract
1/2 cup unsweetened apple sauce

Instructions

Preheat the oven to 350 degrees.

In a small saucepan over low heat, melt the margarine and add in the sugar. Stir until the sugar is dissolved.

Grease and flour a 10-inch spring form pan. Pour the margarine/sugar mixture evenly into the bottom of the spring form pan. Then place the pineapple rings on top of the margarine/sugar mixture. Place a cherry inside each ring.

In a mixing bowl, combine the flour, sugar, baking powder and salt. Add in the canola oil, almond milk, apple sauce and vanilla extract. Stir until everything is well-combined.

Pour the batter into the spring form pan. Bake for 50-60 minutes, until a toothpick inserted in the dough comes out clean.

Remove from oven and slide a knife around the outer edge of the cake pan. Let cool completely before removing the cake from the pan.

Gently turn the pan onto a serving platter, lift off the pan and serve.

Lemon Cake

Never been a fan of lemon cake, to be honest. But this one is for all the Sansa lovers out there. (Sorry, I couldn't resist the *Game of Thrones* reference.)

Ingredients

For the cake:

3 Tbsp lemon juice (about 2 large or 3 small lemons)

2 Tbsp lemon zest

1 1/2 cup all-purpose flour

1 cup sugar

1 tsp baking soda

5 tbsp canola oil

1 tsp apple cider vinegar

1 tsp vanilla extract

3/4 cup water

For the Icing:

2 Tbsp lemon juice

3/4 cup confectioners sugar

Instructions

Preheat oven to 350 degrees and grease a bread loaf-sized baking dish.

Make the cake

In a large mixing bowl, combine flour, sugar and baking soda and whisk until well-combined.

In a separate bowl, combine lemon juice, water, oil, vanilla extract and vinegar. Whisk until combined.

Now add the lemon juice mixture to the bowl of dry ingredients and whisk until well combined. Do not over-mix.

Pour the batter into your prepared baking dish and bake for 25 minutes, or until a toothpick inserted in the cake comes out clean.

Remove from oven and set aside to cool for at least a hour or so.

Make the icing

Combine 2 Tbsp of lemon juice with the confectioner's cigar and whisk until well-mixed.

When the cake has completely cooled, spread the icing over the top of the lemon cake. Allow the icing to set, then serve.

Carrot Cake

My mom's favorite cake. If you like, add some little marzipan carrots on top to make this a professional-quality carrot cake.

Ingredients

For the cake

2 1/3 cups all-purpose flour
1 tsp baking powder
1 1/2 tsp baking soda
1 tsp cinnamon
1/2 tsp nutmeg
1/2 tsp salt
6 Tbsp flax seed meal
3/4 cup warm water
1 1/2 cup sugar
1 cup canola oil
1 tsp vanilla
2 cup shredded carrots
1 cup walnuts, chopped

For the frosting

8 oz vegan cream cheese
1/4 cup margarine, softened
1 tsp vanilla
2 cup powdered sugar

Instructions

Make the cake

Preheat your oven to 350 degrees and line two 8-inch square baking dishes with parchment paper, allowing the excess parchment paper to extend over the edge of the dish. We will later use the parchment paper to lift out the cake after it bakes.

In a bowl, combine the flour, baking powder, baking soda, cinnamon, nutmeg and salt. Whisk until well-combined.

In a large mixing bowl, combine the flax seed and water. Whisk in the sugar and oil. Add the vanilla and shredded carrots, and mix again.

Now add in the flour mixture and stir until everything is just combined. Fold in the walnuts, then divide the batter equally between the two baking dishes.

Bake for 18-20 minutes, or until a toothpick inserted in the cake comes out clean.

Remove from oven and allow to cool for 5 minutes. Then lift the cake out by the parchment paper and allow to fully cool, about an hour or so.

Make the frosting

Using a hand mixer, combine the cream cheese and margarine until it is nice and fluffy. Add in the powdered sugar and vanilla extract and mix gently until smooth.

Complete the job

When the cakes have completely cooled, cover with the cream cheese frosting (and add marzipan carrots if you like). Place in the fridge until ready to serve.

Red Velvet Brownies

Combine red velvet with brownies, and let everyone know what an amazing home chef you are!

Ingredients

2 1/4 cup oats

1/2 large cooked beetroot (boil for 20-30 minutes, then peel while still warm)

1/4 cup unsweetened cocoa powder

1/3 cup almond milk

1/4 cup canola oil

1/2 cup cooked black beans, drained and rinsed

1/2 cup maple syrup

1/2 tsp baking powder

1/4 tsp salt

1 tsp vanilla extract

1/2 cup chocolate chips

Instructions

Preheat oven to 375 degrees. Line a 6-inch by 9-inch brownie pan with parchment paper.

In a blender or food processor, combing the oats, cocoa powder, salt and baking powder and blend/process until they form a powdery, flour-like substance.

Then, add in the almond milk, vanilla extract, canola oil and maple syrup and blend/process until everything is well-combined.

Then, add in the cooked beetroot and black beans and blend/process until everything is well-combined and a thick batter has formed.

Stir in the chocolate chips and then pour the mixture into the parchment-lined baking pan.

Bake for 22-24 minutes, or until a toothpick inserted in the brownies comes out clean.

Remove from heat, let cool for 20 minutes, and serve.

Blueberry Crisp

This is a hugely impressive summer dessert dish and is just so darn easy to make!

Ingredients

2 1/2 cups frozen blueberries
2 Tbsp maple syrup
1 Tbsp cornstarch
1 Tbsp fresh lemon juice
1 tsp vanilla extract
1 cup old fashioned oatmeal
1 cup oat flour
1/3 cup coconut sugar
1/4 cup coconut oil, solid state
1/2 cup unsweetened cinnamon apple sauce
1 tsp baking powder
1/2 tsp salt

Instructions

Preheat your oven to 375 degrees and line an 8-inch square pan with parchment paper.

In a mixing bowl, combine the maple syrup, cornstarch, vanilla extract and lemon juice. Fold in the frozen blueberries and stir gently. Set aside.

In a separate bowl, combine oatmeal, oat flour, coconut sugar, baking powder and salt. Stir in apple sauce, then coconut oil. This will serve as the dough for your crisp. Take half of the dough and press into the bottom of the prepared pan.

Then pour your blueberry mixture evenly on top of the dough.

Pour the rest of the dough mixture on top of the blueberries.

Bake for 40 minutes, or until the top crumble is light brown in color.

Let cool a bit and serve.

Peach Cobbler

Another baked fruit dessert dish. Use fresh peaches in season and you will be delighted by the results.

Ingredients

1/2 cup sugar

2 Tbsp cornstarch

4 cups sliced peaches

1 cup water

Ground cinnamon

1 cup whole wheat pastry flour

2 Tbsp sugar

1 1/2 tsp baking powder

1/4 tsp salt
3 Tbsp margarine
1/2 cup soy milk

Instructions

Preheat oven to 400 degrees.

In s saucepan, combine sugar and cornstarch and stir. Add in 1 cup of water and peaches and bring to a boil. Turn off heat and stir for 1 minute.

Pour mixture into a greased baking pan and sprinkle cinnamon over the top.

In a separate bowl, combine flour, sugar, baking powder and salt. Fold in the margarine and stir until well-combined. Add soy milk and stir well.

Drop this flour mixture in spoonfuls evenly over the peaches. (There should be gaps in the covering, which will spread upon baking.)

Bake for 25-30 minutes, until top pieces are light brown.

Let cool and serve.

Chocolate Mousse

I could eat gallons of chocolate mousse, especially since this is so easy to make.

Ingredients

1 12 1/3-ounce package silken tofu
3/4 cup almond milk
1 cup chocolate chips
1 tsp vanilla extract

Instructions

Place almond milk and chocolate chips in a microwave-safe bowl and heat in the microwave for about a minute, or until melted. Stir until you have a nice rich chocolate milk. Set aside to cool.

In a blender, combine the chocolate milk, tofu and vanilla extract and blend until smooth. Taste and determine if it needs more chocolate. If so, melt some more chocolate chips and toss in the blender.

Pour out into 4 small bowls or ramekins, and chill in the fridge until the mousse sets, about 2 hours. Serve.

Tiramisu

I had no idea that you could make a vegan tiramisu until I tried it. So here you go, get it done!

Ingredients

Ladyfinger cookies
2 cups all-purpose flour

2 tsp baking powder
1 tsp baking soda
1/2 cup margarine
1 cup sugar
1/3 cup maple syrup
1/2 cup almond milk
Tiramisu
1 1/2 cups soy cream cheese
1 1/2 cups soy sour cream
3/4 cup powdered sugar, sifted
2 cups strong brewed coffee, cooled to room temperature
2 Tbsp Marsala wine
2 Tbsp unsweetened cocoa powder

Instructions
Make the ladyfingers
In a large bowl, combine the flour, baking powder and baking soda and stir until well-mixed.
In a separate bowl, use an electric hand mixer to cream together the margarine and sugar until it is nice and fluffy. Stir in the maple syrup and almond milk.
Add the margarine-sugar-milk mixture to the bowl of dry ingredients and whisk until

well-combined. Cover and place in the fridge for an hour.

Preheat your oven to 350 degrees and line two baking sheets with parchment paper.

Remove the dough from the fridge and roll the dough into 1-inch balls. Then roll each ball into a 2-inch by 1-inch rectangle. Place the cookies on the baking sheets and bake for 8-10 minutes, until the cookies are golden-brown.

Remove the cookies from the oven and let cool on the baking sheet for a couple of minutes, then transfer to a wire rack to completely cool.

Make the tiramisu

In a mixing bowl, use a hand mixer to combine the cream cheese, sour cream and powdered sugar until well-mixed.

In a shallow bowl, combine the coffee and wine.

Take a ladyfinger and dip in the coffee-wine mixture for a few seconds until soaked through on both sides, then place in a 5-inch by 9-inch baking dish. Make one layer in the baking dish using about 8 ladyfingers.

Take your cream cheese mixture and spread half of it over the top of the ladyfingers in the baking dish.

Make another layer of coffee- and wine-soaked ladyfingers and then cover with the remaining cream cheese mixture.

Cover the dish and place in the fridge for at least one hour.

Remove from the fridge, dust with cocoa powder and serve chilled.

Chocolate Açaí Bowl

This dessert isn't even bad for you. You could even eat this one for breakfast. It's full of antioxidants and delicious healthiness (yes, that's a word).

Ingredients

1 frozen açaí packet

1 banana

1 Tbsp unsweetened cocoa

1 Tbsp maca powder

1/4 cup almonds (or any other nut/seed you like)

1 tsp agave nectar

1 cup of almond (or any other non-dairy) milk

2 cups of ice

Toppings: blueberries, chopped strawberries, ground peanuts, sliced banana, mango, cacao nibs, shredded coconut

Instructions

Place ice on the blender and pulse until crushed.

Add in the remaining ingredients (except for the toppings) and blend until smooth.

Place mixture in a bowl and top with whatever toppings you like! (Some of my favorites are listed above.)

Banana Pudding

Easy to make, hard to put away. The bananas give this dish a real fresh taste, great for spring or summer.

Ingredients

1/3 cup sugar

4 Tbsp cornstarch

1/8 tsp salt

3 cups coconut milk, divided

1 1/2 tsp vanilla extract

3 very ripe bananas, sliced

48 vegan vanilla wafer cookies

Instructions

In a small saucepan, combine sugar, cornstarch and salt and whisk until combined. Whisk in the coconut milk and then bring the mixture to a boil. Then turn heat to low and simmer for 5 minutes, until the mixture has thickened.

Stir in the vanilla extract and banana slices.

Line the bottom of an 11-inch by 7-inch baking dish with half of your wafer cookies. Pour the pudding on top, covering the entire layer of cookies. Then place the remaining cookies on top, cover the dish with plastic wrap and chill in the fridge for an hour.

Serve chilled.

Chocolate Dessert Shake

I love a good dessert shake. This one incorporates dates for a extra kick of sweetness.

Ingredients

2 cups almond milk

2 frozen bananas

4 dates

1/2 tsp ground cinnamon

2 Tbsp unsweetened cocoa powder

Optional toppings
Soy whipped cream
Chocolate syrup
Chocolate chips

Instructions

Place all ingredients (except toppings) in a blender and blend until smooth.

Top with optional toppings and serve immediately.

Vanilla Cashew Shake

Get some good vitamins and protein in this recipe, which, as a bonus, tastes just like a vanilla milkshake!

Ingredients

1 banana
1/3 cup raw cashews
1/3 cup non-dairy milk (I use
unsweetened, original flavor almond milk.)
1 Tbsp maple syrup
1 Tbsp chia seeds
1/2 tsp vanilla extract
Pinch of salt
1 cup ice cubes

Instructions

Okay this one is easy. Put everything in your blender and blend until smooth.

Pumpkin Pie

Pumpkin pie, the best pie in my opinion (please, no hate mail). This is a simple and effective recipe.

Ingredients

For the crust

1 1/2 cups all-purpose flour, plus additional for rolling

1 Tbsp granulated sugar

1 Tbsp white vinegar

Fine salt

1/2 cup coconut oil

4 Tbsp ice water

For the filling

One 15-ounce can of pumpkin puree

8 ounces silken tofu

2/3 cup granulated sugar

2 Tbsp cornstarch

1 tsp ground cinnamon

1/2 tsp ground nutmeg

1/2 tsp vanilla extract

Fine salt

Instructions

Make the crust

Combine the flour, sugar, vinegar and 1/2 tsp salt in a food processor, and pulse to combine. Add in the coconut oil a spoonful at a time, until a crumbly dough forms. Add in 4 Tbsp of ice water, and pulse the mixture until well-combined.

Wrap the dough in plastic wrap, and press into a 1/2-inch thick slab, and place in the fridge for at least two hours.

Remove the dough from the fridge and let it get back to room temperature. Roll the dough into a 12-inch disc on a flour-dusted surface. Lay the dough carefully onto a 9-inch pie plate, folding the edges under itself, and crimping the edges around the plate. Chill in the fridge for 30 minutes.

Preheat the oven to 350 degrees.

Place some foil in the pie crust and fill with pie weights (or use dried beans or rice if you don't have pie weights). Bake for 20-25 minutes, until the edges are just barely golden. Remove the foil and pie weights, and continue to bake for another 15-20 minutes, or until the crust is barely golden all over. Remove from the oven and place on a wire rack to cool.

Make the filling

In a blender or food processor, combine the pumpkin, tofu, sugar, cornstarch, cinnamon, nutmeg, vanilla extract and 1/4 tsp of salt. Blend/process until completely smooth.

Make the pie

Pour the filling into the pie crust, and bake for 40-45 minutes, until firm. Remove from the oven and cool on a wire rack, until completely cool. Chill in the fridge for at least two hours.

Slice and serve.

Deep Dish Apple Pie

Ah, Americana. Act like a true vegan American, and bring this to your next harvest festival or Thanksgiving dinner.

Ingredients

For the dough

3 cups all-purpose flour, plus some for rolling

2 Tbsp granulated sugar

2 Tbsp white vinegar

Fine salt

1 cup coconut oil

8 Tbsp ice water

For the filling

4 pounds of mixed apples
2/3 cup granulated sugar, plus some for sprinkling
2 Tbsp fresh lemon juice
4 Tbsp coconut oil
3 Tbsp all-purpose flour
1 tsp ground cinnamon
1/4 tsp salt
2 Tbsp unsweetened almond milk

Instructions

Make the dough

Combine the flour, sugar, vinegar and 1/2 tsp salt in a food processor and pulse unit well-combined. Add in the coconut oil slowly, and pulse until the largest pieces are the size of a pea. Add in the ice water and pulse again, until everything is evenly combined.

Divide the dough into two equal parts and cover in plastic wrap, forming each part into 1/2-inch discs. Place in the fridge for at least an hour.

Make the filling

Peel, core, and cut the apples into 1/2-inch thick slices. Toss immediately with the sugar and lemon juice in a large bowl. This will keep the apples from browning.

Melt the coconut oil in a large pan over medium heat. Add in the apples and cook about 10 minutes, or until the apples are softened but not mushy.

Add in the flour, cinnamon and 1/4 tsp of salt, and stir. Remove from heat and let the mixture cool completely.

Assemble the pie

Remove the dough from the fridge and let come to room temperature (this should take about a half hour).

On a floured surface or parchment paper, roll the first disc into about a 13-inch disc, and place into the bottom of a 9 1/2-inch deep-dish pie pan.

Carefully pour the cooled filling into the pan.

Roll the other dough disc into a 12-inch disc and place on top of the filling, crimping together the two pieces of dough at the edges.

Brush the top and sides of the dough with almond milk, and sprinkle sugar all along the outside. Make some decorative cutouts in the top piece of dough, so that steam will be able to escape and not damage the crust.

Refrigerate for at least one hour.

Preheat oven to 425 degrees and place a baking sheet on a rack in the lowest possible position in your oven.

Place your pie pan on top of the baking sheet and lower the oven to 375 degrees.

Bake until the outside of the pie is golden, about 60-70 minutes.

Remove from the oven and let the pie cool for at least 2 hours before serving.

Sweet Potato Pie

Another great pie, as the good old versatile sweet potato is perfect for a warming fall dessert.

Ingredients

For the crust

1/2 cup pecans, coarsely chopped

1/2 cup rolled oats

1 cup whole wheat pastry flour

1/4 cup coconut oil

2 Tbsp maple syrup

For the filling

3 Tbsp cornstarch

3/4 cup dark brown sugar

2 sweet potatoes, peeled, boiled for 20 minutes and allowed to cool

3/4 cup unsweetened almond milk

1 tsp nutmeg

1 tsp cinnamon

1/2 tsp sea salt

Instructions

Make the crust

Preheat oven to 375 degrees.

In a blender, combine pecans and oats and blend into a powder. Combine this mixture with the flour and whisk until they are combined.

Add in the coconut oil and whisk until well-combined.

Stir in the maple syrup and mix well again. You should have a dough-y type of texture right now.

Transfer the mixture to a 9-inch pie pan and press into the bottom and sides until even all around the pan. Poke a few holes in the bottom and sides of the pan.

Bake for 20-25 minutes, or until the crust is lightly golden brown.

Remove crust from the oven and allow to completely cool.

Make the filling

In a large mixing bowl, combine the brown sugar, cornstarch and whisk until combined. Add in the sweet potato, almond milk, nutmeg, cinnamon and salt and whisk again until everything is well-combined.

Bake the pie

Pour the filling mixture into the cooled crust.

Bake for about one hour, or until the filling is just set at the edges.

Let cool for an hour, and serve.

Pecan Pie

Yet another fall pie, this one has always been a classic in my family. The pecan halves baked into the top of your filling give this one an extra bit of class.

Ingredients

For the pie crust

1/4 cup margarine, chilled and cut into cubes

1/4 cup vegan shortening, chilled and cut into cubes

1 1/2 cups all purpose flour, plus some for rolling
1/2 tsp salt
1 Tbsp sugar
5 Tbsp ice water
For the filling
1 Tbsp coconut oil
1 1/2 cup pecan halves
1/2 tsp ground cinnamon
1 cup sugar
1/2 cup maple syrup
1/4 cup margarine
2 Tbsp flax meal + 6 tbsp warm water
10 salted crackers, crushed
1 Tbsp flour
1 1/2 tbsp vanilla extract

Instructions

Make the crust

Combine margarine, shortening, sugar, flour and salt in a food processor and pulse until the largest pieces are pea-sized. Pour in the ice water and mix until just combined.

Form the dough into a 1/2-inch thick disc. Wrap in plastic wrap and chill in the fridge for an hour.

After the hour is up, preheat your oven to 325 degrees. Remove the dough from the fridge and roll out until it is 1/4-inch thick. Gently place the dough in your pie pan and shape it to fit the pan. Crimp the edges if you like, and poke holes in the bottom and sides with a fork. Place aluminum foil just around the edges so that they do not burn.

Bake for 10 minutes, and remove from the oven.

Make the filling:

On a large skillet, melt your coconut oil over medium heat. Add in the pecans and stir until coated in coconut oil. Add in cinnamon and continue stirring until the pecans are fragrant and just lightly toasted (Don't burn them!). Remove the mixture from the pan and place in a bowl. Pick out a 1/2 cup of the nicest pecan halves to place on the top of the pie, then roughly chop the remaining 1 cup of pecans.

In a small bowl, whisk together the flax meal and water and set aside for 5 minutes, until they gel together.

In a small saucepan, combine the sugar, maple syrup, margarine, flax meal mixture, crackers, flour and chopped pecan pieces. Heat over medium-low heat and stir until the mixture has thickened, about 5 minutes.

Remove from heat, stud in the vanilla extract, and pour the mixture into the prepared pie crust. Make sure the edges of the pie crust are still covered with aluminum foil, and bake for 30 minutes. Remove foil from the edges of the crust, and place the pecan halves carefully on top of the pie in a decorative pattern. Bake another 10-20 minutes, or until the filling is set on the edges but not quite set in the middle.

Remove from oven and set aside to cool. Serve warm or at room temperature.

About the Author

Sidney Griffin is author of several cookbooks on Vegan diet. He has written research papers on the topic and currently lives in California.

www.ingramcontent.com/pod-product-compliance
Lightning Source LLC
LaVergne TN
LVHW011956070526
838202LV00054B/4943